Gluten Free For Beginners

Go Gluten Free and Maximize Your Health and Longevity

Jim Berry

Table of Content

Important Insight

It is not often that a medically prescribed diet goes mainstream attracting millions of followers many of whom are not even suffering from the health conditions for which the diet is normally prescribed. Certainly, the *gluten free diet* is one of these diets– if not the only medical diet of its kind to become a successful and sensational dieting craze. In fact the gluten free rage has become so popular that it gave birth to a new, robust, and fast expanding gluten free processed food industry.

The gluten free diet is a specifically formulated diet prescribed by doctors to people who are suffering from the Celiac disease as well as those with gluten intolerance. This diet is the only known medical intervention for these ailments. It cannot be considered a cure as it does not in any way eliminate the celiac disease or make gluten sensitivity go away for good.

The diet merely relieves the symptoms and makes the conditions highly manageable allowing the patients to live normal lives. Both the celiac disease and gluten intolerance are not really life threatening but they are downright distressing and cuts your productivity tremendously.

The problem with celiac and gluten intolerance is they are often either misdiagnosed or left undiagnosed for a long time because of the similarity of their symptoms to many other equally distressing health conditions. Add to that, if left untreated, these conditions can lead to more serious and really life threatening conditions like cancer and other autoimmune disorders that can wreck havoc to your whole system.

Under normal circumstances, it takes about 4 to 6 years before a patient is finally confirmed to have the celiac. This is because celiac diagnosis requires an invasive biopsy procedure to confirm its presence - and doctors are not likely to perform such unless the patient's condition is serious enough to justify the procedure. Instead, the doctors go through trial and error rigmaroles to rule out the existence of other conditions with similar symptoms.

They will normally prescribe medications for these other conditions first and observe - *a negative response for which means it is not likely to be the cause of the symptoms*. They would do this over and over again forward guessing the underlying condition until either the symptoms subside or become worst enough for them to order a biopsy. More often than not, by the time the doctors order a biopsy, the celiac disease has progressed to a point that secondary conditions have developed making the whole scenario more complicated and extremely difficult to manage.

How it came to be a diet rage adopted not only by people at risk but by millions of non-sufferers as well should not be surprising at all. In the first place, there is now a growing awareness on the celiac disease and the many ramifications it has on their lives.

Celiac disease is an inherited autoimmune disorder where the autoimmune system produces an anomalous, destructive response for people afflicted with the disease. The presence of gluten in the digestive system triggers the autoimmune system to attack the walls of the small intestines to destroy the finger like structures called villi which are responsible for absorbing nutrients from the food we eat into the bloodstream. Once the villi are destroyed, the body's ability to absorb much needed nutrients is gravely impaired leading to more serious autoimmune disorders, osteoporosis, unexplained infertility, some neurological conditions, and in a few cases, even cancer.

Gluten intolerance (*or gluten sensitivity*) is also a gluten induced condition that is almost identical to the celiac disease. People who have this condition manifest the same symptoms of a celiac disease. However, in this case, the destructive autoimmune response to the presence of gluten is not triggered and the walls of the small intestines are not destroyed. The patients in this case are simply intolerant to gluten and their bodily responses can be linked more to an allergic reaction much like lactose intolerant people react to milk. Health authorities are however still investigating whether or not prolonged gluten intolerance will ultimately lead to celiac.

Initial interest for the gluten free diet naturally came from celiac sufferers (*whose numbers could easily reach 3 million*) and the gluten intolerant (*estimated at 18 million Americans*) including an undetermined number of others who suffer from simple wheat allergy. If you are to consider the fact that many of those afflicted with the celiac disease are asymptomatic (*and therefore left undiagnosed*) plus the fact that both celiac and gluten intolerance are almost always misdiagnosed, you would hardly credit the above numbers as being responsible for triggering the gluten free dieting rage and giving birth to a new, multibillion dollar gluten free processed food industry. The numbers would be intermittent and won't be enough though to start a frenzied dieting rage.

What really triggered the gluten free dieting craze were the numerous and well publicized testimonials by quite a number of famous celebrities attesting to the beneficial effects of the diet - more prominent of them is pop singer Miley Cyrus who even exhorted her more than 4 million Twitter followers to go gluten free like her. With celebrity endorsements appearing left and right on entertainment tabloids complete with their before and after pictures showing their slim figures as proof of the diet's efficacy, it was a matter of time before scads of their non-celiac and non-gluten-sensitive followers followed suit giving birth to a $5 billion gluten free processed food industry.

With 2/3 of the American population said to be either obese or overweight, the gluten free diet is like a breath of fresh air for many of them and the much publicized celebrity endorsements of the gluten free diet becoming seemingly like bolts of lightning - sparking a fiery and spontaneous response from a receptive audience already primed to pounce on anything that will give them relief for their weight problems.

And before one can say Jack Robinson, gluten free became synonymous with good health and weight loss - to the consternation of some health experts who were quick to point out (*albeit, correctly*) that simply eliminating wheat, barley, and rye from the diet will not result in weight loss. However, food manufacturers were quick to recognize the opportunity and were even quicker in filling supermarket shelves with newly concocted processed gluten free food items. People remained undaunted by warnings of health authorities, saying the gluten free diet will only benefit the celiac sufferers and those with gluten sensitivity. Just the same, they continued to line up the counters with their gluten free product purchases.

The whole gluten free craze has also triggered an ongoing debate among health and dietary experts on whether or not the gluten free diet can really lead to weight loss. Admittedly, the claim that simply replacing wheat, barley and rye with other non-gluten containing grains will not lead to weight loss - in fact, in some cases it may even lead to the individual gaining weight. They cite the sugar laden gluten free processed foods that started to flood the supermarkets as example.

However, what the gluten free diet detractors are missing is the fact that there can be an ideal gluten free diet which is not solely about eliminating gluten. In other words, the diet doesn't have to be merely gluten free, it can also be low carb and high protein at the same time. Sad to say, however, most if not all of the processed foods labeled 'gluten free' which you will find in the supermarkets are far from ideal. They are not only sugar laden but are also loaded with simple starch that can cause spikes in blood sugar levels.

The ideal gluten free diet must also be a *low carb, high protein* diet derived from unprocessed food sources that are as natural and organic as they can be. By this definition, the ideal gluten free diet effectively eliminates all processed foods (gluten free or not) from your shopping list – which as will be explained later, ultimately leads to significant weight loss. This is what you will learn as you go through the rest of this book. The book is about developing the ideal, well balanced, gluten free diet that will help individuals shed weight without the need of counting calories.

1: It is in the Food We Eat

Most of what the ailments of modern man comes from the food he eats today. The respected authorities in the field of gluten free diet agree to the fact that modern grain is slowly killing us and leading to illnesses that could have been avoided by simple lifestyle changes. They also have observed one sad thing about the food industry – it is run by people who do not give a hoot about the public's health. Instead, what we have is a profit driven food industry that continuously mislead the public by selling them foods that they made people believe as nutritious but are in fact wrecking havoc to their health.

What is basically wrong with modern Western diets?

Since man inhabited the planet, he had been subsisting on a natural *low carb, high protein, gluten free diet* sourced mostly from the wild plants and animals he was able to forage, gather or hunt from his surroundings. For millions of years (*before the advent of agriculture and the dawn of industrial age*), man had been consuming the same low carb, high protein, gluten free diet - so much so that the human genome and human metabolic reactions are believed to have practically been programmed to respond favorably only to this type of diet.

Unfortunately, after man discovered agriculture and learned how to grow plants and domesticate wild animals for food, his normal nutritional intake (*to which his bodily functions have been accustomed to respond for millions of years*) was drastically altered or modified causing countless adverse reactions which were totally unexpected. Eventually, mounting documentary evidence started pointing to the contemporary diet (*spawned by modern agriculture and processed with newly found industrial know how*) as the culprit behind the many illnesses (*which has become known as the 'diseases of civilization'*) afflicting man today.

It was only a little over 15,000 years ago when man started acquiring and developing his agricultural skills to produce high yielding agricultural crops and genetically modifying them to make them resistant to pests and pesticides. It took less time than that when man first learned how to prepare and process various food so they can be stored for a long time and used conveniently if and when the need arises. It would be wishful thinking to expect that our bodies will immediately and favorably accept and adapt to the change 0ver to a grain dominated, sugar loaded diet without expecting any adverse reactions. Replacing the low carb to high carb and high protein to low protein plus loading it with refined sugar which was totally alien to the body prior to the agricultural era should only make you expect for the worst. 15,000 years is not long enough to reprogram the human genome to fit the contemporary Western diet without triggering some adverse reactions.

The typical contemporary Western diet contains no more than 15% protein whereas for millions of years our bodies have been programmed to a diet that has 19% to 35% protein. Grain and refined sugar which high glycemic loads are the main source of carbohydrates of modern diets whereas the carbohydrate sources during the gluten free pre-agriculture era came from non-starchy fruits and vegetables which are not only low in carbohydrates but also rich in fiber.

Today's contemporary diets rely heavily on processed and fast foods both of which make use of hydrogenated vegetable oils. It is a normal process in modern food production to hydrogenate vegetable oils to produce cheaper saturated fats which are more economically ideal for large scale food processing. Unfortunately, the hydrogenation process produces trans-fats which not only increases the level of bad cholesterol (LDL) in the blood but also lowers the level of good cholesterol (HDL) putting the person who eat these trans fat containing foods at constant risk of developing cardio vascular diseases and having a heart attack.

Processed foods practically dominate every aspect of modern man's diet and lifestyle. He has in fact become so dependent on processed foods that he can't prepare a meal without them. The sad part is food manufacturers process food so they will have longer shelf lives to make them last long enough until they are bought. As a consequence, you will find processed food with up to ten times more sodium in them to make them last longer. They are high in sodium but low in potassium which puts those who eat them at risk of having high blood pressure, a stroke, or other cardio-vascular diseases.

We live in a world where the food manufacturing industry is run by people who are totally unconcerned with people's health. The main concern of these giant agro industrial corporations is to produce profits for their company. Since it was easier and more convenient for them to feed a growing and hungry population with foods that are also easy to produce, they produce grains and cereals in abundance and through clever marketing tactics turned them into the staple of modern diets.

To their great advantage, the Standard American Diet (SAD) is now sadly dominated by grains and cereals.

As a consequence, this has created a very nasty situation where:

- 2/3 of American adults aged from 20 and above are either overweight or obese

- More than 64 million Americans suffer from some form of cardio vascular disease

- 11 million Americans have type 2 diabetes

- 50 million Americans suffer from hypertension

- 25% die of cancer - 1/3 of these cases are linked to nutritional factors.

The magnitude and scope of the illnesses and diseases attributed to the modern diet has alarmingly increased over time. The cause is in the food we eat and the solution can be as simple as a lifestyle change. If we are to put weight on the evolution of man, 15,000 years is simply not enough time for man to adapt to such a dramatic diet change.

2: It is not just about Gluten

Few people actually realize that modern grains wheat, barley, and rye we consume today are actually genetically modified and fertilized with nitrates to give a higher yield and be more resistant to pest and pesticides. Higher yield means more profits for the producers. Unfortunately, it means having far more gluten than the original wild grass our ancestors used to consume. It also means having more allergenic compounds than the original wheat. Modern wheat for example has been genetically modified from the 14 chromosome wild grass it used to be to a 42 chromosome variety it is today.

The ideal gluten free diet for weight loss however should not be focused merely on eliminating gluten from the diet but on totally eliminating all traces of wheat and other similar grains including rye and barley from the food we eat. This is because they contain *obesogens* or chemical compounds that are foreign to the body and disrupt the endocrine system wrecking havoc on the normal course of development of lipids and balance metabolism causing one to become obese or overweight.

Here are the *obesogens* found in wheat:

- *Gliadin*

  Gliadin is a protein found in wheat and other similar grains belonging to the genus Triticale. Once in the digestive system, gliadin is reduced to polypeptides that easily attach to the opiate receptors of the brain. But instead of relieving pain or stimulating euphoria, the gliadin-derived polypeptides *stimulate appetite*. *Gliadin* also increases the permeability of the small intestin which results in increased water retention further aggravating weight gain.

- *Amylopectin A*

  This is a highly digestible, "complex" carbohydrate found only in wheat and related grains. Their presence creates spikes in blood sugar levels obliging high blood insulin levels which eventually lead to insulin resistance followed by the growth of inflammatory fat.

- *Wheat germ agglutinin*

  This is the carbohydrate binding protein of wheat which has the tendency to bind to the leptin receptor. It is basically an enzyme inhibitor and inhibits the hormone of satiety meaning you will keep on eating without feeling satisfied.

Then again, the ideal gluten free diet for weight loss must not only be about gluten and wheat, but must also eliminate other food items and substances that are foreign to body and causes allergies.

Some of these food items you must avoid include:

- ***Dairy Products***

  Dairy products like milk and butter are modern day food concoctions. They are relatively new on the human timeline. They contain lactose and casein - two substances that cause allergies or severe immune reaction in man. 3 out of 4 people (or 75%) are known to be intolerant to dairy products. Most adults are unable to break down casein and lactose which results in allergies and sensitivities.

- ***Sugar***

  Refined sugar has no nutritional value at all except for its high glycemic load which can cause immediate spikes in the blood sugar levels as they are easily absorbed into the bloodstreams. Unfortunately a large portion of contemporary diets is made up of refined sugar. One third of the calories that are derived from carbohydrates in the contemporary Western diet come from sugar. On the average, Americans consume about 156 pounds of sugar a year or roughly equivalent to 31 bags of five pounders.

- ***Potatoes*** (***except sweet potatoes***)

  They are starchy foods that breakdown easily into sugar and cause spikes in blood sugar levels. They may also contain the glycol-alkaloid toxin called *Solanine* which irritates the gastro-intestinal tract and cause gastro-enteritis.

Avoid the 'Frankenfoods' too

These giant agribusiness interests have practically taken a strangle hold on us by making us totally dependent on the so-called *'Frankenfoods'* or genetically engineered food products which they have produced. Hoodwinking us into believing they are totally safe and feeding health authorities with questionable safety studies, they have practically flooded the consumer market with food products using genetically modified food sources they have created in their labs.

Genetically-modified foods have taken over much of our food supply without us being aware of it. They are used as ingredients in producing processed foods or as feeds for grain-fed cattle the end products of which find their way into our dining tables through the meat we eat along with the artificial genes they have created.

The sad part is despite the claims of the manufacturers and the shady endorsements by health authorities that they are relatively safe for human consumption, an increasing number of independent research studies persistently link the genetically modified foods to the high incidence of allergies, sterility, infant mortality, childhood illnesses, organ defects, and even cancer.

If you don't have any idea of what 'Frankenfoods' are, below is a short list of the more popular ones that has become very much a part of our daily existence.

- ***Genetically Modified Alfalfa***

   If you think you are not consuming Alfalfa, read closely. The natural Alfalfa is an important forage crop cultivated for use as livestock fodder. Since the Romans and the Greek era, Alfalfa has been used by farmers to feed their cows. They have however been genetically modified by giant agri-business interests like Monsanto so that they can produce higher yield and at the same time be resistant to herbicides such as Round up (*a popular herbicide used by farmers to kill the weeds*).

The genetically modified Alfalfa with its transgenes (*artificial genes*) and the herbicides sprayed on them gets into our system through the meat and dairy products we eat. The kind of damage they can wrought to our system is simply unimaginable. Even in its natural form, Alfalfa is known to contain *phytoestrogens* which are basically estrogen blockers that cause reduced fertility in mammals. The Alfalfa seeds meanwhile contain the amino acid canavine which interacts with another amino acid arginine resulting in the synthesizing of dysfunctional proteins which are toxic to humans and produce lupus-like symptoms.

- **Aspartame**

More popularly known as *Nutrasweet*. This is a popular artificial sweetener used in most food processing applications including beverages. Aspartame has been established as a neurotoxin which disrupts brain functions and our immune systems. Despite endorsements by nutritionists and health authorities to its safety, there is mounting evidence that shows that aspartame aggravates insulin sensitivity and causes a lot of other health disorders. In fact one comprehensive study even linked leukemia and non-Hodgkin's Lymphoma to continued aspartame consumption.

- ***Ranch-raised Beef***

The main reason why a Gluten Free lifestyle favors organic meat from pasture-raised, grass fed livestock is because ranch-raised live stocks are fed not only with genetically modified alfalfa but also with genetically modified corn and soy meal. They are also injected with all sorts of things like growth hormones, antibiotics, and vaccines to ensure their health and faster growth. Unfortunately, they also find their way into our bodies through the meat we eat.

- *Canola Oil*

  Almost 90% of the canola produced in the world has been genetically-modified too in order to weather the effects of herbicides (*particularly glyphosate more popularly known as Round Up*) during planting. Aside from the transgenes, large quantities of the herbicide can be found in the finished canola oil products.

- *Corn, corn meal, and Corn Starch*

  With almost all the corn planted in the U.S. being genetically modified to resist herbicides and pesticides, you can be sure that all the products and ingredients made from modified corn carry trans genes too as well as traces of the pesticides and herbicides used. The gory part is genetically modified corn products are used in almost all processed and packaged foods. These include Corn oil, corn flour, corn starch, corn syrup, corn meal, gluten, and sweeteners such as fructose, dextrose, and glucose. They are used in making baked goods, fried foods, snack foods, confectionery, special purpose foods, edible oil products, and soft drinks.

- *Vitamins*

  Take a second look at the vitamins you are taking. They may have been manufactured from genetically modified plant sources or may have used genetically modified ingredients as carriers. For example, Vitamin C is usually made from *Frankencorn* while vitamin E is made from *Frankensoy*.

- *Enzymes*

  Almost all the enzymes used for food processing come from genetically modified products like the enzymes used to prevent egg products from spoiling; enzymes that removes the bitter taste from beer; enzymes that improve the clarity of fruit juices; enzymes to help milk clotting for making cheese; enzymes to speed the rise of bread dough; and enzymes used to manufacture many food supplements.

- *Ice Cream*

  One thing you should be wary of when you buy ice cream is whether or not it contains several genetically-modified ingredients like corn starch, high fructose corn syrup, and milk from cows that were injected with bovine growth hormone (rBGH). The bovine growth hormone is injected into cows to make them grow faster and produce more milk. In studies made on rBGH by the University of Vermont as commissioned by agribusiness giant Monsanto, five calves were born from cows injected with rBGH with rare deformities that were never seen before. This was however downplayed. Can you imagine if rBGH filters into your system from the ice cream you eat?

- ***Infant Formula***

  Manufacturers of infant formula who used frankenfood ingredients like genetically modified soy and milk from rBGH injected cows may be unmindful of the health hazards they bring. You should be wary of this before you buy your next infant formula.

- ***Margarine and Shortening***

  Contrary to the general belief margarine and shortening made from vegetable blends and canola are not healthy. Most of the ingredients used are genetically modified.

- *Milk*

  Milk from cows injected with bovine growth hormone (rBGH) may contain blood and pus as a result of infection resulting from the rBGH injection. Studies have shown that cows injected with rBGH become highly susceptible to infections and those which becomes infected may have blood and pus in their milk along with the rBGH and any antibiotics that may have been injected into the cows to prevent the spread of the infection.

- *Soy and Lecithin*

  Almost all of the soybean crops planted are genetically modified soy which means all soy products including Lecithin may have harmful trans genes. Lecithin is normally used as a thickener by food processors and packaged food manufacturers.

- *Sugar Beets*

  Most sugar beets from which 35% global supply of refined white sugar come from are also mostly genetically modified. So, you not only risk having a spike in your blood sugar levels but also the risk having artificial genes filtered into your system along with fertilizer, herbicide, and pesticide residues.

- **Tomatoes**

  Tomatoes have been genetically modified so they will have longer shelf life. They have a reversed DNA sequence so that they won't soften even if stored longer. They however have much less nutrients than organic tomatoes on top of the modified genes they pass on to us.

- **Vegetable Oil**

  Most if not all the "vegetable oil" sold in supermarkets are refined from genetically modified soybean oils, canola, corn, or cotton seed.

3: Why the Gluten Free Diet is Ideal for Weight Loss

There are so many weight loss diets that are in existence today. They come as fast as they go – many of them failing miserably to achieve sustainable weight loss for their followers. For the gluten free diet however, it is quite apparent that it is here to stay if we are to base it on the interest people continue to shower on it – which makes people wonder why the gluten free diet is effective for weight loss while others are not.

Conventional wisdom tells us that people get fat or gain weight because of the energy imbalance that goes in and out of your system. If you have more calories than what the available fat cells can handle then the body will create more fat cells to store the excess calories. In other words, if the energy you burn is equal to your energy intake then your weight is likely to remain constant. If your energy intake is more than the energy you burn then you are likely to gain weight. If you burn more energy than what you take in, you are likely to lose weight. You are likely to end up over-weight or obese over time if you continue to consume more calories than you burn.

There are also mitigating factors that may abet or hasten weight gain like:

- An active/inactive lifestyle
- Unhealthy environment
- Eating habits
- Genes
- Hormone imbalance
- Medication
- Age
- Emotional state
- Pregnancy
- Lack of Sleep
- Smoking

These factors makes you predispose to eating more food than your body can burn and most weight loss diets are built solely around the principle that by taking in less calories than you can burn you'd be able to prevent fat build up and lose weight in the long term. This simplistic approach to weight loss, while perfectly correct, is leaving an important factor to chance.

Fat cells are not produced by the body merely to store carbohydrates for fuel for later use. Fat cells are also produced by the body to temporarily house toxins which the liver is unable to filter out -

particularly when there is too much toxins for the liver to handle at any given time.

The capacity of the liver to filter out wastes and toxins is limited. As long as there are more toxins than the liver can handle, fat cells are created where the toxins are diluted in water and stored until such a time when the liver can finally attend to them and filter them out. In other words, the body's first line of defense against toxins is the fat cell. This is how our system ensures there won't be too many toxins in the blood to poison us.

It also means that no matter how much and how long we starve ourselves of carbohydrates by dieting, we won't be able to gain much ground and lose as much weight as we want if our bodies continue to be bombarded with toxins. At best, we'll only lose weight during the course of our dieting only to gain back whatever weight we shed once we stop dieting.

The gaping hole that allows toxins to get into our system must be plugged to help the liver get rid of toxins that are already inside our systems. Otherwise, the liver will be tied up with old toxins that continue to build up and start causing damage thus affecting their metabolic capabilities.

Where do the toxins come from and how do we plug the gaping hole?

Toxins and other poisonous substances foreign into our bodily system through the food we eat, through the water we drink, and even through the air we breathe. They come in various forms from toxic residues of antibiotics injected into livestock and poultry to fend off diseases, from the growth hormones they are fed to insure their growth, from the industrial feeds produced from genetically modified corn meal and grains.

They get embedded in the meat of the farm animals we buy from the supermarket. They can come in the form of fertilizer, herbicide, and pesticide residues that remain in the farm produce such as fruits and vegetables. They can come in the form of high concentrations of sodium and sugar in the water we drink and the processed foods we purchase. Toxins may also come in the form of environmental pollutants in the air we inhale.

What happens is the endothelial cells lining the walls of our blood vessels communicate directly with the newly formed fat cells and instruct them to store the toxins diluted in water to keep the blood clean of toxins. If the fat cells are metabolized, the toxins will be released into the bloodstream.

However, our immune system will prevent the breakdown or metabolism of these fat cells if the amount of toxins embedded in them will compromise our health once these toxins are released into the blood stream. This is the reason why some people have difficulty losing weight despite starving themselves almost to death by dieting.

The only way to plug the gaping hole and prevent further toxin build up in our bodies is to eat only natural, unprocessed, gluten free foods. This will give the body enough time to rest from the influx of more toxins than the liver can possibly handle allowing more elbow room to rid the body of whatever toxins are already inside. This is basically what the gluten free diet is all about and the very reason why it is more superior to other dietary regimens for weight loss.

Sustainable weight loss is a natural side effect of going gluten free. The gluten diet is able to naturally shed those extra pounds without difficulty simply by focusing on an eating regimen that gives the body some respite from the onslaught of toxins.

4: The Ideal Gluten Free Food Guide

To get your gluten free diet into gear, you need to have a clear cut idea on which food contains gluten. That will mean anything that is derived from or makes use of wheat including all the grains that belongs to the genus Triticale like barley and rye. The idea is to be able to identify them on site and get rid of them before they can contaminate other food stuff.

This should not be a problem though because 4 out of the 5 major food groups are naturally gluten-free namely fruits and nuts, vegetables, meat, and dairy products. Just make sure you get them fresh and unprocessed meaning as close to their natural form as possible. For meat, poultry, and fish, make sure they are organic. The meat and poultry products should come from pasture-raised, grass-fed live stocks and free of antibiotics or growth hormone injections. The fish must not come from fish farms but caught instead from the wild. Fruits, nuts, and vegetables must be organically grown and free of fertilizers, herbicides, and pesticides.

The only difficulty you may encounter is in ferreting out the 'stealth gluten' especially from processed food ingredients. Food manufacturers try all possible tricks they can think of to disguise gluten containing ingredients on their food labels and if you are not careful and vigilant your efforts to go gluten free will amount to nothing.

To get you started, here is a partial list of gluten free foods you can include in your shopping list:

Main Food Groups	Grains and Starches
<ul><li>Fresh meats, poultry, and fish (not breaded, marinated, or batter-coated)</li><li>Unprocessed beans, nuts, and seeds in their natural form</li><li>Fruits</li><li>Fresh vegetables</li><li>dairy products (with the exception of some)</li><li>Fresh eggs</li></ul>	<ul><li>Gluten-free flours (rice, soy, corn, potato, bean)</li><li>Rice</li><li>Corn and cornmeal</li><li>Quinoa</li><li>Sorghum</li><li>Buckwheat</li><li>flours made from rice, corn, potato, soy, bean</li><li>Amaranth</li><li>Flax</li><li>Arrowroot</li><li>Millet Flour</li><li>Tapioca</li><li>Teff</li></ul>

What you need to avoid in general are food and drinks that may contain Wheat (*and other products derived from it like Durum flour, Bulgur, Farina, Kamut, Graham flour, spelt, and Semolina*), Barley (*and other products derived from it like malt, malt flavoring, and malt vinegar*), triticale, and Rye.

Foods to Avoid

• Breads made from Wheat, barley, or Rye	• Beer
• Cakes, pastries, and pies	• Soups and soup bases
• Cookies and crackers	• Croutons
• Cereals	• Gravies
• Processed luncheon meats	• Candies
• Imitation meat or seafood	• Seasoned snack foods
• Canned vegetables	• French fries
• Self-basting poultry	• Salad dressings
• Pastas	• Seasoned rice mixes
• Sauces, including soy sauce	
• Matzo	

Speaking of 'stealth gluten', here a list of food you must avoid because they may have hidden gluten in them:

- Pickled foodstuff that used malt vinegar - The vinegar is made from barley.

- Canned Black-eyed Peas – They are made with hydrolyzed wheat protein.

- Root Beer – It uses modified food starch which contains gluten.

- Shredded Cheese –Wheat flour is usually added to the cheese to keep them from sticking together.

- Curry Powder – Wheat flour is used here to prevent the curry mixture from clumping.

- Mouthwash – It uses grain alcohol which contains gluten.

- Non Stick Cooking Sprays – It uses grain alcohol too as propellant.

Ingredients that contain gluten

Abyssinian Hard Barley malt, Bread flour Broth Cereal (including extracts and binding) Edible starch Farina Flour (all-purpose,) Horderum vulgare Kamut Malt beverages Malt syrup, , and Malt flavoring Oats Rye Semolina Vital gluten Wheat Wheat germ oil	Avena (wild oat) Barley extract Beer, other fermented beverages Couscous Durum Filler Flour (bleached) Germ Hydrolyzed wheat protein Malt extract Malt vinegar Matzo Oriental wheat Oat bran, Oat syrup Rice malt Spelt Wheat berry Wheat starch	Bouillon Blue Cheese Bulgur Croutons Einkorn, wild einkorn Flour (bleached) Gluten, Glutenin Hydrolyzed oat starch Malted milk Mustard powder MIR (wheat, rye) Oat fiber, Brown rice syrup Sprouted wheat Triticale Seitan Wheat bran Whole wheat berries	Barley (Hordeum Vulgare) Bran Dinkle Emmer, wild emmer Flour (enriched) Fu Graham Flour Hydrolyzed wheat gluten Maltose Miso Oat gum, Soy Sauce Udon Tabbuleh Wheat gluten Wheat germ Wheat grass

Gluten-Free Ingredients

Adipic Acid Acacia Gum (gum Arabic)	Acetic Acid Annatto Beta Carotene	Aspartame BHA Brown Sugar	Algin Baking Yeast Brewer's Yeast

Benzoic Acid	BHT	Cream of Tartar	Caramel Color
Carrageenan	Calcium	Carob Bean Gum	Corn Syrup Solids
Carboxymethyl	Disodium EDTA	Ethyl Maltol	Fumaric Acid
cellulose	Dextrose	Gelatin	Guar Gum
Cellulose	Glucose	Karaya Gum	Lactose
Fructose	Lactic Acid	Maltol	Maltodextrin
Invert Sugar	Malic Acid	Methylcellulose	Psyllium
Lecithin	MSG –	Polysorbate 60; 80	Stearic Acid
Mannitol	monosodium	Sucralose	Sodium
Pectin	glutamate	Sodium Benzoate	Metabisulphite
Propylene Glycol	Papain	Tartaric Acid	White Vinegar
Sucrose	Sorbitol	Vanillan	Yeas
Sodium Nitrate;	Sugar	Xylitol	
Nitrite	Tartrazine		
Titanium Dioxide	Tragacanth		
Vanilla Extract	Yam		
Xanthan Gum			

5: Maintaining a Gluten Free Lifestyle

Embracing a gluten-free lifestyle is a tough row to hoe. It requires a lot of determination and is therefore not for the faint of heart. Most people get discouraged as they transition from their old lifestyle to a gluten free lifestyle basically because of the many pitfalls and temptations along the way. A lot of them do not know where to begin while others who were able to get a jump start gets lost or waylaid along the way.

For one thing, gluten is often used as a food binder and you can be almost sure the food manufacturers will never admit they actually used gluten for their products labeled gluten free. The trickiest part is unearthing these 'stealth gluten' intentionally omitted by manufacturers from the food labels. This is basically the main reason why it is extremely difficult to maintain a truly gluten free diet. You are up against food manufacturers who are more concerned with the profit they can squeeze from you than your health.

Here are some tips and tricks on how to maintain a gluten free lifestyle:

- Search vigilantly for 'stealth gluten'. Look for them too in beverages, readymade sauces and packaged powdered gravies, and even in some spices.

- When you're not sure, skip it. This should be your guiding principle always. It is always better to skip food you are not sure contains gluten.

- Arm yourself with more knowledge about gluten and their sources so that you'd be able to easily identify their presence anytime anywhere. Be familiar with the funny names used by food manufacturers to conceal the gluten content in their food products. Strive be a complete label reader.

- When attending parties or social gatherings where food is served, make it a point to inquire about the ingredients. It is prudent not impolite to inquire. And if you think the food served contains gluten, decline it in a nice manner without offending the host.

- Be wary and vigilant of possible cross-contamination. Make sure the cooking vessels used to cook gluten loaded foodstuff were not used to prepare gluten free meals.

Turn your Kitchen into a Gluten Free Zone

Keeping your kitchen gluten free isn't really that difficult although it does require more attention and care. Here are some tips on how to get started:

- Throw out all gluten-containing foods and anything that may have been contaminated.

- Clean all kitchen surfaces and all cooking equipment well.

- Throw away wooden utensils and cutting boards and anything else that has porous surfaces. They may have trapped gluten containing particles in the pores. Give away any kitchen equipment that cannot be completely cleaned of gluten like a bread toaster.

- To avoid possible contamination, buy condiments in squeeze jars.

6: Your 7-Day Gluten Free Diet for Weight Loss

A typical balanced gluten free meal to achieve an effective and lifelong weight loss should at least look like this:

- Must have 4 to 8 ounces of lean meat for protein (like lean beef, pork loin, turkey, chicken, or seafood). 30%

- Multiple servings of differently colored vegetables for carbohydrates (raw, lightly cooked, or steamed). 40%

- Complete it with healthy fats from any of these – olive oil, avocado, almonds, macadamia, pecans, or walnuts. 30%

The recommended calorie intake ratio of every balanced gluten free meal should be 40% Carbohydrate, 30% Fat, and 30% Protein. An easy way to make sure you get the right fill is to get a plate and fill it with ½ to 2/3 full of fruits and vegetables and the rest of the plate with your choice protein source and favorite healthy fats.

Of course this is something that is not written in stone. This is merely a guideline which you can change to suit your personal preference or specific needs. There is also no need to count calories as long as you stick to a low carb, high protein regimen.

A balanced gluten free meal plan will bring back the hormonal balance and condition your mind and body to "want" to lose weight. Basically, your appetite will be tempered and your cravings reduced.

Below is a 7 Day Gluten Free Balanced Diet Plan for weight loss.

	Breakfast	Lunch	Dinner	Snacks
First Day	Apple and Chicken Sausage	Chili Pulled Pork	Gluten Free Meat Loaf	Beef Jerky
Second Day	Gluten Free Breakfast Casserole	Quick Ground Pork Lunch	Bacon and Tomato Quiche	Pumpkin Seeds
Third Day	Green Monster Smoothie	Chili Maple Pork Chops	Mango Avocado Spiced Chicken Salad	Gluten Free Granola Bar
Fourth Day	Bacon Fritata w/ Kale and Mushrooms	Chicken Dippers	Beef Stew w/ Squash Butternut and Kale	Apples and Almond Butter
Fifth Day	Spicy Stew w/ Poached Egg	Coconut Honey Chicken	Bacon and Tomato Quiche	Bacon and Guacamole Sandwiches
Sixth Day	Egg Muffins	Stir Fry Beef	Hunter Stew	Baked

		Teriyaki		Cinnamon Apple Chips
Seventh Day	Smoked Salmon, Dill, and Red Pepper Scramble	Beef Broccoli with Cashew Nuts	Grilled Tri Trip	Cauliflower Popcorn

7: Your Gluten Free Breakfast Recipes

Day 1 Chicken Apple Sausage

1 pound ground chicken
1 peeled finely diced apple
1 tbsp fresh finely chopped thyme leaves
3 tbsp finely chopped parsley, fresh
1 tbsp finely chopped oregano, fresh
2 tsp garlic powder
Salt
Pepper
Coconut oil

Instructions:

- Preheat oven to 425^0F.
- Place a skillet on a medium to high heat and pour three tablespoons of coconut oil.
- Add in the finely diced apples, finely chopped thyme, finely chopped parsley, and finely chopped oregano and cook for 7 to 8 minutes or until the apples are softened.
- Remove from the heat and place in one corner to cool for five minutes.
- Stir in the ground chicken together with the pepper, salt and garlic powder.

- Form 12 half inch thick patties from this meat mixture and arrange well in a baking tray that has been lined with tin foil.

- Place inside the oven and bake for twenty minutes.

- Cool and store in a refrigerator or freezer.

- Microwave for a few minutes or pan fry in coconut oil until browned.

- Serve hot.

Day 2 Gluten Free Breakfast Casserole

1 lb. breakfast sausage, removed from their casings
1 sweet potato, large , diced
2 to 3 cups of chopped baby spinach
1 green onion, diced
10 to 12 eggs, large
Sea salt
Ground pepper

Instructions:

- Preheat oven to 375^0

- Grease a glass baking dish (9"×13") with coconut oil.

- Heat a skillet over medium to high heat.

- Stir in the sausage and cook until browned and totally cooked through.

- Remove the cooked sausage from skillet but retain the sausage grease.

- Add the diced sweet potatoes to skillet and stir cook for ten to fifteen minutes or until the sweet potatoes are tender.

- Remove the sweet potatoes from the skillet and place in a bowl.

- Add in the sausage, spinach, green onion, sausage, pepper and salt. Mix until all the ingredients are well combined.

- Place the mixture in the greased baking dish making sure they are spread out evenly.
- Place the eggs in a separate bowl and whisk. Pour evenly the whisked egg over the sausage and veggie mixture in the baking dish.

- Place inside the oven and bake for twenty five to thirty minutes or until the mixture has set. Cool slightly and cut into squares before serving.

Day 3 Green Monster Smoothie Breakfast

1 cup coconut milk
1 cup of spinach leaves
1 cup of kale
1/2 cup of cubed fresh pineapple
1 banana, frozen
1/2 cup of water
1/2 cup of ice cubes
Optional:
1 tbsp coconut butter
1/4 tsp ground cinnamon
1 tsp honey

Instructions:

- Place the coconut milk in first in a food blender place and add the rest of the ingredients.

- Pulse the mixture until smooth.

Day 4 Bacon Frittata w/ Kale and Mushrooms

For the pesto:
1.5 cups basil leaves, packed
1.5 tablespoons garlic, minced
½ teaspoon rock salt, finely ground
¼ teaspoon pepper
¼ cup of olive oil
3 tablespoons pine nuts
For the frittata:
5 pieces bacon
1.5 cups of kale, chopped
2 small zucchinis, cut into spirals
1 cup of button mushrooms, sliced
½ teaspoon garlic powder
6 pieces eggs, beaten
Black pepper, cracked

Instructions:

- Preheat oven to 375^0.

- Place a large skillet on medium heat and fry the bacon until slightly crispy. Place on a plate lined with paper towel and set aside.

- Scoop out most of the fat from the bacon leaving just one tablespoon of it in the skillet.

- Add the sliced mushrooms and cook for two minutes. Stir in the kale, garlic powder, and zucchini noodles. Cook until most of the kale has softened or wilted.

- Pour in the eggs evenly over the noodles. Season with enough pepper and cook for two minutes until the eggs have set on the bottom.

- Place inside the oven for twenty to twenty five minutes. Stick a knife through the middle of the frittata and if it comes out dry and clean then it is done.

- While the frittata is still in the oven, start to prepare your pesto sauce.

- Put all of the Pesto ingredients inside a food processor and pulse until the mixture is creamy. Adjust the taste to your liking by adding seasonings.

- Serve the frittata hot from the oven together with the basil pesto on the side.

Day 5 Spicy Stew w/ Poached Egg

2 finely chopped chicken sausages
4 pieces chopped crispy bacon,
1½ teaspoon olive oil, extra-virgin
1 sliced onion
A handful of spinach
1 can tomatoes, organic, diced
2 tablespoon tomato paste
½ cup chicken stock
1 teaspoon chili powder
½ teaspoon smoked paprika
1 clove garlic
A dash of sea salt
A dash of pepper, freshly ground
½ teaspoon red pepper flakes
3 pieces organic eggs
2 teaspoons vinegar

Instructions:

To make the Stew:

- Heat oil in a medium-sized pot and sauté garlic.

- Add in the sliced onions and sauté for five more minutes or until the onions are translucent.

- Stir in the finely chopped chicken sausage and stir-cook until the sausage is cooked thoroughly

- Microwave or fry the bacon until they are crisp. Pat off the excess fat and set aside.

- Stir in the chicken stock, diced tomatoes, spices, and tomato paste into the pot and combine well.

- Add the spinach and reduce the heat into a simmer

To make the Poached Egg:

- Boil three cups water and add in one dash of vinegar

- Crack one egg into the ramekin.

- Just before the water starts boiling, swirl the water with spoon.

- Drop the egg slowly into the boiling water.

- Spoon out the poached egg and place over stew. Serve with the crispy bacon on the side.

Day 6 Egg Muffins

1 tablespoon of olive oil
1 finely chopped sweet onion, large
1 finely chopped green pepper
1 finely chopped red pepper
1 finely chopped jalapeno pepper
12 pcs large eggs
1/2 teaspoon black pepper
1/2 teaspoon salt

Instructions:

- Preheat oven to 35^0 F

- Grease a frying pan with olive oil and place over medium to high heat.

- Sauté onions for 2 to 3 minutes over medium-high heat in then add all the finely chopped peppers. Stir cook for another 2 to 3 minutes.

- Remove the sautéed peppers from the heat and cool.

- Whisk the 12 pieces of eggs in a large mixing bowl. Stir in the cooled sautéed peppers and mix well.

- Add more pepper and salt & pepper if necessary.

- Grease a large muffin tray with coconut oil. Fill each muffin cup with 1/4 cup of the egg mixture.

- Place inside the pre-heated oven and bake for ten to fifteen minutes or until the tops are fluffy and golden brown.

- Remove from the heat and pop out each muffin with a sharp knife.

- At your option, you may garnish each muffin with guacamole, chipotle, or some salsa before serving.

Day 7 Smoked Salmon, Dill, & Red Pepper Scramble

2 whole eggs
1 egg yolk
2 pcs smoked salmon
1 tbsp finely chopped fresh dill
⅛ tsp garlic powder
⅛ tsp red pepper flakes
Pepper
Salt
1 to 2 tbsp coconut oil

Instructions:

- In a large bowl, whisk the two eggs then add the torn salmon and the finely

- chopped dill together with the red pepper flakes, garlic powder.

- Sprinkle with some salt and pepper to suit your taste and mix well.

- Place a small saucepan on low heat and add coconut oil.

- Add the egg mixture to the hot sauce pan and stir cook with a wooden spoon until the eggs are completely cooked.

- Top with roasted vegetables and sweet potato wedges before serving.

8: Your Gluten Free Lunch Recipes

Day 1 Chili Pulled Pork

2 lb pork roast (trimmed of fat)
3 cloves garlic
½ cup of hot sauce
3 tbsp paprika, smoked
2 tbsp chili powder
2 tbsp garlic powder
1 tbsp cumin
2 tsp cayenne pepper
1 tbsp red pepper flakes
2 yellow onions, diced
1 yellow bell pepper, diced
Salt
1 red bell pepper, diced
2 cans of tomatoes, fire roasted
1 can tomato sauce, (14 ounce)
Avocado slices for garnishing
Diced green onions for garnishing

Instructions:

- Poke 3 holes into the pork roast with a knife in 3 different spots. Insert 1 clove of garlic into each hole.

- Place the pork roast inside a crock pot.

- Pour all the hot sauce over pork roast making sure it is well covered all over.

- Sprinkle the top of the pork roast with chili powder, paprika, cumin, garlic powder, red pepper flakes, cayenne pepper, and salt.

- Place the tomatoes, the bell peppers, diced onions, on top of the pork roast and pour the tomatoes sauce all over the roast.

- Close the crock pot, set it on low and cook for eight to ten hours.

- Garnish with chopped green onions and avocado slices.

Day 2 Quick Lunch Ground Pork

1 sweet potato
2 pcs bacon
10 pcs asparagus, chopped, ends removed
¾ lb Italian sausage
½ avocado, sliced thin
Salt

Instructions:

- Preheat oven to 425^0.

- Poke the sweet potato all over with a fork. Wrap with a tin foil and place inside the oven and bake until soft (45 minutes to 1 hour).

- Keep the baked potato wrapped in tin foil so it will stay warm.

- Cook the bacon in a large pan on medium heat until crispy. Set the cooked bacon pieces on top of paper towel to drain any excess fat.

- Sauté the asparagus for five minutes using the rendered bacon fat remaining in the pan.

- Add the Italian sausage and break it up using a wooden spoon. Continue to sauté until the meat is well cooked.

- Cut the baked potato in half and place in 2 separate bowls.

- Top each half of the baked potato with meat, bacon, avocado and asparagus.

Day 3 Chili Pork |Chops w/ Maple Syrup

1 tsp red pepper, ground
½ tsp chili powder
1 tsp garlic powder
½ tsp cayenne pepper
⅛ tsp black pepper
¼ tsp salt
2 tbsp coconut oil
2 half pound pork chops sliced thin, with the bone in
3 tbsp maple syrup
¼ cup of orange juice
1 tsp apple cider vinegar
Green onions for garnishing

Instructions:

- Place the ground red pepper, the chili powder, the garlic powder, the cayenne pepper, salt, and the black pepper and mix well in a small container.

- Pat dry the half pounder pork chops with a cloth or paper towel.

- Sprinkle each side of the pork chops with the mixed seasoning making sure the seasonings are pressed into each side of the pork chops.

- Place a large pan over high heat and add the coconut oil.

- Add the pork chops to the now hot pan. Sear each side of the pork chop for 2 to 3 minutes each.

- When done, turn down the heat to low.

- Whisk together the apple cider vinegar, the maple syrup, and the orange juice then pour into the pan all over the pork chops.

- The mixture will thicken and start to bubble. Leave the pork chops to cook for another 6 to 8 minutes, flipping once to make sure each side is well coated with the thick sauce.

- Remove the pork chops from the heat and place in a serving plate together with the remaining sauce. Arrange the chopped green onions on top before serving.

Day 4 Chicken Dippers

1 lb skinless, de-boned chicken breast
1 egg
½ cup of almond flour
1 cup shredded coconut
Salt
Coconut oil
Maple Mustard Sauce (for use as dipping)

Instructions:

- Preheat oven to 350^0.

- Cut the chicken into strips.

- Whisk the egg in a shallow bowl. In a separate bowl, combine and mix the coconut, almond flour, and salt.

- Dip the chicken strips one by one - first in the whisked egg bowl then in the coconut mixture. Make sure all sides are well coated. Place the coated chicken strips on a plate.

- Place one to two tablespoons of coconut oil in a large pan on medium heat and wait until it is hot enough.

- Add the chicken strips into the pan making sure they are not crowding each other.

Cook the chicken strips in batches for about one minute on each side.

Arrange the cooked chicken strips on a cooling rack and place the rack atop a baking sheet.

Place the baking sheet inside the pre-heated oven for 10 to 12 minutes until the chicken strips are cooked through.

Cool the baked chicken strips on the rack. Once cooled, dip each strip into the maple mustard sauce and serve.

Day 5 Coconut Honey Chicken

To make the rice:
1 small cauliflower crown, cut into florets
⅓ cup of chicken broth
¼ tsp salt
1 tsp garlic powder

To make the honey chicken:
1.5 lbs chicken thighs, cut into 1" cubes
1 to 2 tbsp coconut oil
Salt

To make the sauce:
2 tbsp coconut oil
2 cloves garlic, minced
1 can of coconut milk (14 ounce)
½ yellow onion, small, minced
¼ cup of honey
½ cup of coconut aminos
½ tsp red pepper flakes
2 to 3 tbsp sriracha
Salt
¼ cup of tapioca flour
Green onions chopped for garnishing

Instructions:

- Shred the cauliflower florets with a food processor until it resembles rice.

- Place a saucepan or a Dutch oven over medium heat until hot.

- Add the cauliflower rice, garlic powder, salt, and chicken broth. Cover and let steam for ten minutes while stirring once in a while to prevent the mixture from sticking to the bottom of the pan.

- Place a separate saucepan over medium heat.

- Pour in some coconut oil and wait until it is very hot.
- Add the chicken cubes to the pan, sprinkle with salt and sear. Make sure to flip over the chicken cubes when they begin to turn white so as to cook the other side.

- With a slotted spoon, after chicken has cooked through, remove with a slotted spoon and set aside.

- Add two more tablespoons of coconut oil to the pan (if necessary) then sauté the onion and garlic until the onion turns translucent.

- Stir in the sriracha, coconut milk, coconut amines, honey, salt, and red pepper flakes. Stir cook together until it comes to a low boil then reduce the heat to low.

- Stir in the tapioca flour one half at a time while whisking to make sure it is fully incorporated into the mixture. Don't stop whisking or the tapioca flour will start to clump.

- Add the cooked chicken cubes once the mixture to thicken.

- Cook for at least one minute to make sure the chicken cubes are reheated.

- Pour the chicken together with its sauce on top of the cauliflowers rice. Arrange the chopped green onions on top before serving.

Day 6 Stir Fry Beef Teriyaki

2 tbsp coconut oil
2 cloves garlic, minced
½ cup of coconut aminos
1 tsp grated ginger, fresh
3 tbsp honey
1 tbsp Sriracha
½ tsp fish sauce
1 tsp sesame oil
2 tbsp arrowroot powder
1 red bell pepper, sliced thinly
1 bell pepper, sliced thinly
½ yellow onion, sliced thinly
1 cup button mushrooms, sliced
1lb thinly sliced flank steak
Salt
Pepper
Green onions, chopped for garnishing

Instructions:

- Place a large pan over medium heat.

- Add coconut oil sauté the minced garlic together with the grated ginger.

- Once the garlic aroma comes out, turn the heat to low.

- Stir in the coconut aminos after the pan has cooled down a bit. This will prevent the aminos from splattering.

- Slowly increase the heat to medium then add the fish sauce, sesame oil, sriracha, and honey.

- Bring the mixture into a slow boil, then add half of the arrowroot powder in small batches at a time while whisking to make sure they incorporate well into the sauce.

- Once the sauce has thickened, add the mushrooms, the onions, and peppers. Simmer for six to eight minutes until the onion turns translucent.

- Remove the cooked vegetable and place in a bowl.
- Increase the heat to medium-high then add the flank steak slices. Cook the meat slices for 2 to 3 minutes on each side until the pinkish color of the meat is gone.

- Toss in the cooked vegetables and stir until well combined with the meat.

- Add the remaining one tablespoon of arrowroot again a little at a time at a time while whisking to make sure the powder is fully incorporated with the mixture.

- Place the chopped green onions on top before serving.

Day 7 Beef Broccoli w/ Cashew Nuts

1 cup of coconut aminos
3 tbsp honey
½ cup orange juice
1 tsp fish sauce
1 tsp grated fresh ginger
2 cloves garlic , minced
½ tsp red pepper flakes
3 tbsp arrowroot powder
1 lb thinly sliced flank steak
3 broccoli crowns cut into florets
Salt
Pepper
2 tbsp of coconut oil
½ cup cashews, toasted

Instructions:

- In a large bowl, combine the coconut aminos, arrowroot powder, honey, orange juice, ginger, fish sauce, red pepper flakes, and garlic. Season with pepper and salt and whisk together.

- Place the flank steak slices in a shallow dish and pour the whisked mixture to cover the meat slices.

- Marinate for thirty minutes inside the refrigerator.

- Place a Dutch oven on medium heat and add one tablespoon of coconut oil.

- Add the cauliflower florets when the Dutch oven is hot enough.

- Season with some salt and stir fry until soft and crisp.

- Remove from heat once the broccoli is cooked to your preference.

- Place the Dutch oven back over high heat.

- Add more coconut oil then place the meat slices together with the marinade and cook until the meat slices are no longer pinkish in color.

- Add back the cooked broccoli florets together with the toasted cashews.

- Simmer for one more minute then serve hot.

9: Your Gluten Free Dinner Recipes

Day 1 Gluten Free Meat Loaf

1 1/2 lbs ground beef
1 tbsp Worcestershire sauce
1 can tomato sauce, (4 ounce)
1/3 cup fried pork skins, crushed
2 eggs
2 1/2 tbsp chili powder
1 tbsp garlic salt
1 tbsp garlic pepper seasoning

Instructions:

- Preheat the oven to 375 degrees F.

- Combine the ground beef, tomato sauce, crushed pork skin, Worcestershire sauce, and eggs in a large mixing bowl.

- Season with garlic pepper, then with chili powder, and then with garlic salt.

- Mix until the mixture is well blended. Form the mixture into a loaf and place in a previously greased loaf pan.

- Place inside the oven and bake for thirty five to forty minutes.

- Leave it out to rest and cool for at least five minutes.

- Slice the roast into serving pieces when cool enough.

Day 2 Bacon & Tomato Quiche

For the Zucchini Hash Crust:
2 small zucchini, organic, grated
1 1/2 tablespoon coconut flour
1 egg, beaten
1 tablespoon coconut oil
1 teaspoon flax meal
1/8 teaspoon sea salt

For the Quiche:
5 eggs, beaten
1/2 cup egg whites, organic
3 tablespoon plain almond milk, unsweetened
5 slices cooked organic bacon, chopped
2/3 cup cauliflower, ground into rice
1/2 cup chopped spinach, fresh
1/4 teaspoon mustard, ground
1/4 teaspoon sea salt
1/4 teaspoon black pepper

For the topping:
2 small sized tomatoes, sliced
1/2 cup cheese of your choice, grated

Instructions:

- Preheat oven to 400 F.

- Wrap the grated zucchini in cheese cloth and squeeze over the sink to drain the liquid out of the zucchini. Place the drained zucchini in large mixing bowl.

- Add all the rest of the crust ingredients to the zucchini and mix well.

- Place the zucchini mixture into previously greased pie dish. Use the back of a spoon to spread the zucchini mixture evenly around the pie dish until the dish is fully covered with the zucchini crust mixture.

- Place inside the oven and bake for nine minutes to form the crust.

- Take out the pie crust from oven and place in one corner for a while.

- Combine the eggs, almond milk, egg whites, ground mustard, black pepper and sea salt in a large bowl.

- Add the chopped bacon, cauliflower rice, and chopped spinach to the egg mixture and mix well.

- Pour the egg mixture into zucchini crust to form the quiche.

- Arrange the tomato slices on top of the quiche and return inside the still hot oven.

- Bake for twenty minutes checking at the twenty minute mark to make sure the edges of the pie crust is not browning too much.

- Place a sheet of parchment paper loosely to cover the top of the pie dish before returning it to the oven.

- Put the pie back into the oven once more and bake for the remaining eight minutes, or until the top is browned and center of the pie is firm and set.

- Add the cheese on top and return inside the oven back into the oven to bake for two minutes more.

- Remove and allow to cool. Slice and serve.

Day 3 Spiced Chicken Salad w/ Mango & Avocado

1 small head of lettuce, chopped
1 to 2 cups of shredded chicken
1 medium size mango, peeled and diced
1 avocado, diced
1.2 teaspoon of chili powder
1/2 teaspoon of cumin powder
Salt
Pepper

Instructions:

- Place the chopped lettuce in a large mixing bowl.

- In a separate, medium size bowl, place the shredded chicken and moisten with a little bit of water.

- Microwave for twelve to fifteen seconds.
- Add the cumin and chili powder.

- Arrange the shredded chicken over the lettuce and top with avocado and diced mango.

Day 4 Beef Stew w/ Kale and Butternut Squash

2 tablespoons bacon fat or coconut oil
1 roughly chopped onion
2 pounds of stew beef cut into one inch cubes
1 1/2 tablespoon of minced fresh sage
4 cloves of garlic, minced
4 cups of cubed butternut squash
1/2 teaspoon paprika, smoked
 16 ounces of frozen kale, chopped (you may use 1 bunch of fresh kale)
4 cups of beef stock
Salt
Pepper

Instructions:

- Heat 1 tablespoon of bacon fat or coconut oil in a large Dutch oven over medium high heat.

- Fry the meat in batches until browned but be careful to cook it only half through or slightly browned. Set aside the browned meat for a while.
- Adjust the heat to medium and pour in the remaining coconut oil or bacon fat.

- Once it's hot enough add the smoked paprika, garlic, sage, and onions to the pot.

- Sprinkle with salt and a dash of fresh pepper. Stir fry until the onions turn translucent and are softened. (Around 8 minutes).

- Stir in the beef cubes, kale, and butternut squash to the pot. Combine well with continuous stirring then then pour in the chicken stock. Add two more cups of hot water.

- Allow it to boil first before you put on the cover.

- Reduce the heat and simmer for one hour.

- Serve hot. Store the leftovers in the refrigerator where you can keep it for up to a week.

Day 5 Hunter Stew

Butter
2 pounds beef, cut into cubes
2 handfuls of fresh blueberries
2 cups of young carrots, cut lengthwise in half
Coconut oil
Pepper
Garlic powder
Salt
Oregano
1 large Onion cut thinly in circles

Instructions:

- Stir fry the beef cubes in coconut oil over medium heat until browned. Add in the onions and allow simmer until the onions soften.

- Stir in the young carrots together with the seasoning.

- Add a few drops of Worcestershire sauce plus enough water to cover the meat.

- Bring to a boil and stew on medium heat for thirty minutes until the carrots are fork tender.

- Add the fresh blueberries in the last 10 minutes together with a teaspoon of butter.

Day 6 Grilled Tri Trip

1 beef tri-tip roast (2 1/2 pounds)
1 tbsp salt
1 1/2 tsp garlic salt
1/2 tsp celery salt
1/4 tsp black pepper, ground
1/4 tsp onion powder
1/4 tsp paprika
1/4 tsp dried dill
1/4 tsp dried sage
1/4 tsp dried rosemary, crushed

Instructions:

- Combine the garlic salt, paprika, salt, onion powder, celery salt, dill, black pepper, sage, and rosemary in a mixing bowl. Place inside an airtight container and set aside at room temperature.

- Moisten the roast with a damp cloth then pat with the rub we prepared above. Refrigerate and chill the whole night.

- Set an outdoor grill over high heat and lightly brush the grates with oil.

- Place the roast on the grill and sear until brown on all sides then remove.

- Adjust the grill temperature to medium-low indirect heat and return the roast.

- Grill for one and a half hours, turning the roast occasionally until the desired doneness is reached.

- Remove from the heat and wrap in aluminum foil. Let it rest for ten minutes then carve into thin slices across the grain.

- Serve.

Day 7 Jerusalem Artichoke and Hamachi Carpaccio

2 to 3 pieces of peeled young Jerusalem Artichokes (sunchokes)
¼ pounds hamachi, sashimi grade
Olive oil, extra virgin
Yuzu juice
Tobiko and Shiso for garnishing
Smoked sea salt

Instructions:

- Arrange the thin slices of Jerusalem Artichokes together with the slices of hamachi sashimi in layers.

- Drizzle the top with olive oil and Yuzu juice, then sprinkle with sea salt.

10: A Tapered Approach to a Gluten Free Lifestyle

As we mentioned earlier, the Gluten Free diet is more than a diet. It is a whole new lifestyle. And, you can't simply slip in into a new lifestyle like changing your under wears.

A transition into the Gluten Free lifestyle requires a tapered, slower approach. You have to take one small step at a time to acclimatize your body to the new eating regimen. In the first place our dependence and addiction to sugar and our cravings for everything sweet has been cemented by decades of eating sugar loaded processed foods. It won't go away overnight.

The best way to transition into the Gluten Free lifestyle is to take a tapered approach by taking one Gluten Free meal at a time during the first few weeks until you gradually become adapted to the new eating regimen. It will be too daunting to do it in one big leap. Besides, if you fail on your first try, you are likely to feel so frustrated that you may want to leave the diet altogether out of desperation.

A tapered approach will allow you to gradually adopt the diet over the first few weeks, one meal at a time. This means you won't be doing it all in one go. Doing so is not only daunting but may possibly lead you to failure.

Here is how to transition to the Gluten Free lifestyle gradually within 6 weeks.

Week	What to do	Why you should do it
1	Introduce Gluten Free Breakfasts and start reducing your sugar intake. You can take your regular fare for lunch, dinner and snacks.	Breakfast is the hardest meal of the day to change over to Gluten Free. First, you are always pressed for time to make the preparations. Two, for years now, we've stereotyped breakfasts to bread and cereals and it may seemingly be unimaginable not to have them around anymore. However, just by changing your first meal and avoiding further sugar intake for the rest of the day will help a lot in minimizing the erratic spikes in your blood sugar levels as well as stabilize your energy levels throughout the day. You can have bacon and eggs and bacon for breakfast but skip the breads and the cereals. Have some fresh fruits too, or make a vegetable and fruit smoothie for breakfast. Throw in some mixed nuts for added protein. The bottom line is to make your breakfast Gluten Free for the first week and avoid foods loaded with sugar for the rest of the day. This should break you in to the Gluten Free lifestyle smoothly.
2	Introduce Gluten Free Dinner. You will now have 2 Gluten Free meals for the day.	Now that you've tasted Gluten Free for breakfast, you are ready to add your dinner to the changeover. This means you should not eat anything that is not in your Gluten Free food list after 5 p.m. It will also mean you'll be going to bed with lower sugar levels which will minimize the fat deposits which normally occur at night as you sleep. You may keep your usual dinner recipes but with some modifications and as long as you

		take out the grains, the beans, the dairy, and all processed foods. Instead of rice you can use cauliflower florets mashed into the consistency of rice. Or, you can simply a steak or fish and take a lot of vegetables too.
3	Add the Gluten Free lunch so that all the main meals are now Gluten Free.	This time around all your main meals – breakfast, lunch, and dinner - will be Gluten Free. It will only be your in-between-meals snacks that will remain non-Gluten Free to cater to your now diminishing sugar cravings. Your main meals should however be well planned and your breakfast, lunch, and dinner recipes carefully calendared in such a way that you won't be at a loss on what to prepare when meal time comes around. With lunch now a part of your daily Gluten Free meal plans, the vegetables can play a much bigger role in supplying you with much needed carbohydrates through your lunches. The secret here is to prepare your Gluten Free shopping list based on what Gluten Free foods are available in your area. Then gather all the related Gluten Free recipes together and start stocking up on the needed Gluten Free ingredients. Next, calendar a cooking schedule incorporating each recipe to a date when you wish to prepare them. Consider cooking bigger quantities and using some while freezing the rest for later use.
4 5 6	You are now ready to go 100% Gluten Free for the next three weeks.	By this time, your sugar craving must be gone and doesn't bother you anymore. This means you are ready for the big time and go all out Gluten Free. Your goal for the next three weeks is to totally eliminate everything that is non-Gluten Free which means even your snacks will have to be Gluten Free too. If the pangs of hunger starts biting you between meals, you can snack on nuts, berries, celery sticks, boiled eggs, nut butters, guacamole, and even raw vegetables.

After six weeks, you are likely to fall into one of the 3 categories below:

Category 1:

You achieved significant weight loss, highly energized and have adapted well enough to your new diet to enjoy it.

This means you've struck the perfect nutrient balance for you. The fact that you've lost weight and you are not having any difficulty sticking to the diet only shows your body is getting the right amount of nutrients it needs. You can move on and adopt this diet without further modifications and make it a more permanent lifestyle change.

Category 2:

You may have lost some weight, but your cravings for the foods you've cut out are still nagging and severe. You are also low in energy and you seem to be losing your motivation to continue.

This can mean two things. One, the diet is right for you but your cravings for the foods you missed out is just too powerful. Two, the diet may need a little modifications.

What you can do is create a cheat day within the week. You can stay 6 days on Gluten Free and take 1 day off from it. You may binge on your food cravings on your cheat day. This way, it will help you go through 6 days on Gluten Free since you know that you are coming close to your cheat day when you can splurge on any food you wish. Having a cheat day resets your metabolism on that day which may be good for you in the long term.

Category 3:

You have not lost any weight despite sticking strictly with the regimen for six weeks. Worst, you are not satisfied at all with the Gluten Free food you have been eating.

Having lost no weight at all doesn't mean the Gluten Free diet is not working for you. It's either you have still too many toxins in your body or you haven't struck the right macro nutrient balance yet. What you should do is to stick to the Gluten Free lifestyle and just do some tweaks in your diet.

Try experimenting with different macro nutrient ratios by adjusting the amount of proteins, carbohydrates, and fats in your meal. If you still feel lethargic after making an adjustment then make further adjustments.

Keep on doing it until you hit the right ratio. You'll know you've hit it once you start feeling highly energized and fully satisfied. You should also start losing weight.

You must keep in mind that the Gluten Free diet is a low carbohydrate diet. If for a long time you've been subsisting on a high carb diet, shifting suddenly to Gluten Free may entail bouts of dizziness, lethargy, or constipation. You have to be prepared for this.

Conclusion

I hope this book was able to help you to gain a deeper insight on how best to manage your weight and lose those excess pounds in 7 days by embracing a low carb, high protein Gluten Free Diet. The next step is to put the meal plan into action and adopt the Gluten Free Diet as your lifestyle for the long haul for a healthier, leaner you.

Made in the USA
Middletown, DE
27 January 2023

23326259R00053